Flares, Fatigue & WTF

Wellness Warrior Press

Flares, Fatigue & WTF

Wellnesswarriorpress.com

ISBN: 978-1-990775-65-9

Introduction

If this book landed in your hands, it's because someone you love wants to let you into their world.

Someone with a chronic illness.

What's the purpose of this small but mighty book, exactly? Well, it's very simple: it's intended to help you understand how life feels for someone with a chronic illness. The pain, the guilt, the thoughts—all of it.

It's not always easy for someone with a chronic illness to put their reality into words. By giving you this book, they're saying, "I want you to see me. I trust you with this part of my life."

The fact that you're here, reading these words, shows you care enough to try to understand—and that means the world to the person in your life.

Contents

PAIN, SYMPTOMS & CHAOS

1

It might not show on the outside, but
I often feel like a pile of steaming
horseshit. Whether due to pain,
feeling sick, or being exhausted.

Being inside my body is like being
trapped in a prison cell. There's so
much I want to do, but I can't.

2

Some days, I look happy and move around and get a lot done. I bet that's pretty confusing to see. Especially if I'm bedridden the next day.

My body is basically a crew of greedy creditors that keeps offering me loans only to demand it all back with interest the next day.

So, if I had a good day yesterday and am now paying for it, it frustrates me to hear, "But you looked fine yesterday. What happened?"

I'm already having to deal with the greedy creditors inside my body, and trust me—they're total assholes.

3

Remember when I said I pay for my good days? Sometimes I pay for absolutely no reason, too. Think of it as hidden fees.

And trust me, if I understood why it was happening, I'd do everything in my power to fix it.

Being asked, "What did you do that caused this?" is also frustrating, because it puts the blame on me. As if I could have prevented this. My illness is unpredictable—it can tear me down for pushing too hard, and sometimes, for absolutely no reason.

4

"So, just don't push so hard."

I hear that a lot. And if you felt like death six days out of the week and fairly good one day, wouldn't you want to catch up on things while you're feeling good? Chores? Basic hygiene?

That's what makes this life so difficult.

When I feel close to normal, I want to take advantage of it. Otherwise, I'd live in my own filth and would attract flies. It's not like I'm not going skydiving or bungee jumping, here. I'm maybe catching up on some laundry or tidying my room, or maybe going out for coffee for the first time in months.

I think I deserve that.

5

I constantly get the feeling that people think I'm either lying or exaggerating, because on the outside, I look totally fine.

Do you know how shitty a feeling that is?

Not only do I have to put up with a body that feels like it's decaying from the inside out, but I also have to convince those around me of my truth. Or worse, pretend like I *am* totally fine, especially on my bad days, because I know most people are tired of hearing about it. So, I put on a mask to make others feel more comfortable. And that's also exhausting.

6

Some days, the pain or sickness is so bad that I want to crawl into a hole and die. But I can't—I have responsibilities.

So I push through, even though it feels like it's slowly killing me.

Not because I want to, but because I have no other choice.

Imagine having a nasty flu with body aches and a high fever, but still having to go to work.

That's my life.

7

Having a chronic illness is honestly like being on a rollercoaster with a blindfold. Sometimes your whole body jerks sideways really hard; other times, the ride is smooth. And then out of nowhere, a bee flies into your mouth and you choke.

You never know what's coming next. As much as you want to prepare, you can't.

So I go to bed every night, begging: *Please be okay tomorrow. Or at least, not terrible.*

8

Speaking of symptoms changing, so does my ability to do things.

Some days, I can go for a walk and make myself some food. Other days, something as simple as taking a shower makes my arms burn and gets me totally out of breath and exhausted. And the idea of cooking—I'd rather gnaw on drywall than get up and have to stand for five minutes, even if it's only to heat something up in the microwave.

So even if I did something yesterday, or an hour ago, it doesn't mean I can do it right now.

9

Symptoms can also hit in clusters.

So if I have chronic back pain, well, one day, I might still have my back pain, along with a migraine, numbness in my arms, and skin so sensitive it feels like someone took sandpaper to it all night.

Those are what I call really bad flare days. And those are the days that I need compassion the most—not a whole speech on diet and exercise or an interrogation over my activities the day before.

10

Having a chronic illness is beyond lonely.

Why? Because I barely get to engage in social activities. I either have to cancel the day of because I feel like a baboon's ass, or I'm too afraid to commit because I know I might have to cancel, which puts so much pressure on me that the stress itself can sometimes cause a flare.

GUILT, CANCELATIONS & MISSING OUT

11

I don't want to miss important events.

More than anything, I want to be able to attend. Especially when it comes to birthdays, or ceremonies, or something as big as a wedding day.

When these dates approach, I make every effort to be there. Sometimes, I absolutely do push through, even though it kills me the next day.

So if I can't make it, it's not because I don't care or didn't want to attend.

It's because my body didn't let me.

12

Canceling plans makes me feel like
total shit.

And the worst part? I can often sense
disappointment or irritation from
someone when I cancel on them.

Trust me—I didn't *want* to cancel. I
would have much preferred to be
present with friends and family than
to be at home, either in agony or
tossing around in my own sweat.

I already feel like ass; the anger or
disappointment makes me feel so
much worse.

I imagine it's very frustrating to love
someone who rarely attends
gatherings, but I promise you—I'm not
canceling because I don't care enough
to try. It's torment.

13

Imagine planning to go somewhere very special, only to have to cancel at the last minute. Now repeat this weekly. Maybe daily.

Eventually, you learn that it's better not to make plans at all than to make tentative plans with the possibility of letting someone down.

So instead, I just don't go anywhere. And life gets lonelier.

What would mean the world to me is if someone worked around my illness and agreed to make plans A, B, and C, and if all three didn't work out, would still show compassion and agree to try for plan D or E, if needed.

14

What if I have plans with only myself? Like planning to go pick out a new pair of shoes at a nearby mall?

No one else is involved, right? There's no one to disappoint.

Now repeat this all the time. Wanting to do things, but having to stay home instead, doing nothing other than sleeping, reading, or watching TV.

That's not a very fun life.

It's beyond depressing.

15

The guilt that comes with canceling plans is a nasty feeling.

But you know what's worse? The perception people start to have of you. That you're *flaky. Unreliable.*

When I can't make it somewhere, it has nothing to do with you and everything to do with my body, which is out of my control.

16

"You could at least put in a little effort."

I get it. There aren't many big special days. It's one thing to skip out on a coffee date, and another to miss a family member's birthday party.

What you don't see is that I'm always making an effort. That's just my life. Every day is a struggle.

And the times I do show up—I'm making a huge effort. Every time.

So if I can't make it to an important occasion, it means I'm really not okay, and standing up feels like an Olympic sport.

17

I wish love weren't measured by how many times I show up. Because for me, that's just not sustainable. And it puts so much pressure on me.

I love deeply, even if I can't always be physically present.

18

Guilt sucks.

100%

You know what else does? Grief. It sneaks in after the event—when everyone's raving about how great it was, or when pictures of smiling faces pop up on social media.

And while all that fun was happening, I wasn't living it up at home or dancing to club music.

I was in bed. On the couch. A corpse wrapped in fresh skin.
Missing out on life—yet again.

19

When I miss out on events, I don’t only grieve the actual event, or the time I could have spent with friends and family.

I grieve for the old me. The person who could attend without hesitation, without a week of stress, without the fear of letting everyone down.

I miss that person most of all.

20

You know when you catch a really bad bug? The flu? A stomach virus? The kind that lasts for weeks at a time?

Halfway through, things start to get dark. Not only do you feel like death, but you also miss going out. Doing things. Living life.

Now imagine being told you'll always have this bug, and not having healthy days to look forward to. Being told you won't come out of this.

That's chronic illness in a nutshell. It's emotionally and psychologically devastating in so many ways.

MENTAL
HEALTH

21

Chronic illness is an emotional rollercoaster.

I mourn my old life. How I used to be. Things I used to do that didn't send me into a flare or a crash. And then I get angry at my body because it feels like it's become my enemy.

I'm terrified of what the future holds and am constantly wondering: what if I'm like this for the rest of my life?

22

Because my illness is invisible, I'm constantly being invalidated. People tell me I look fine, or even great, when in reality, I could be feeling like absolute trash on the inside.

Just because I look good doesn't mean I feel good. When people point this out, they may not realize it, but it makes me feel like they're doubting how bad things really are.

23

Constantly missing out on events and outings puts a strain on my relationships. It creates distance between me and the people I care about, which makes me even lonelier and feel even more isolated than I already do.

24

When I'm having a bad day, I do less. I'm mostly sedentary. And that takes a toll on my mental health. It's depressing to sit around the house all day, especially when I look outside and see families going for bike rides or people jogging with music playing through headphones.

I would love nothing more than to just live. Not sit in the darkness of my home and rot because I feel so terrible.

25

Yes, I get angry.

Wouldn't you?

Living in this body is like living with an unreliable roommate. You never know when they're going to trash the place and then expect you to clean it up.

26

Anxiety creeps in more often than I would like, and for so many reasons.

Will I be able to attend a special event that I RSVP'd to? Will my illness progress? Will my partner leave me over this? Will my family abandon me because they're fed up?

The questions are always on my mind.

27

Let's not forget the soul-crushing feeling of being a burden.

Some days, I feel like everyone around me would be happier if I didn't exist, because all I do is disappoint people by not making it to events. Or, I'm just *too much* to handle because I need help to do things I can't do on my own.

28

Doing nothing most days is boring as hell. Sometimes, it's fun to do absolutely nothing—especially when you lead a stressful life and need a break.

Some people think it's easy to sit around and do very little.

Mentally, it's a nightmare. I'm so bored. I want to live. I want to have fun. But my body is a b*tch who gets in the way of everything. I honestly wish we could break up.

29

This is something I don't often talk about, but that's constantly at the back of my mind.

What if I don't even have a chronic illness? What if I have the big C word, and by the time they find it, it's going to be too late for me?

30

I know people are just trying to connect when they try to compare my chronic illness to their aches and pains, but what I go through doesn't go away with rest or after taking some Tylenol.

It really doesn't compare.

And it would be less insulting if there were zero attempts at comparing my lifelong struggle to someone's backache. It feels very dismissive.

MISUNDERSTOOD & JUDGMENT

31

“But you don’t look sick.”

Gee, thanks.

I’ve been working super hard on my corpse-in-disguise aesthetic.

These comments might feel like a compliment to you, but here’s how they're received on my end:

Are you sure you’re sick?
Maybe it’s not that bad.
I don’t believe you.

32

Unsolicited advice.

You mean well—I know.

But trust me, if there's a magic cure out there, I've already Googled it at 2 a.m. and probably wasted money on it, too.

So when you tell me to "just try yoga," or "just drink celery juice," what I actually hear is, "*You're not trying hard enough.*"

Spoiler: I am. And I'm tired of nodding politely like it's the first time I'm hearing this advice.

33

The problem with not looking sick? People expect me to function as if I'm perfectly fine.

If I had two broken legs, you'd cut me some slack. But since you can't *see* what's wrong, suddenly it's on me to explain, defend, and convince you why I can't do whatever it is that needs doing.

34

Compassion usually comes in short waves.

When I first explain my illness, people are sympathetic—until it actually affects them.

A new boss? Patient the first couple of times I miss work. After that, I'm suddenly a "problem employee."

A new friend? Kind at first. But give it time, and I'm the one who "doesn't try hard enough" to keep the friendship going.

35

"What a total hypochondriac."

You think I'm a hypochondriac? A hypochondriac worries when nothing's wrong. But something's clearly wrong, isn't it?

You'd think so, too, if you woke up one day feeling like your butt hole was on fire, and the next day, you couldn't lift your arm without your shoulder sounding like popcorn.

Symptoms come and go—some vanish, others get worse, and new ones pop up just to keep things interesting.

I'm basically a whole circus of WTF's.

36

Judgment doesn't just come from strangers. It comes from friends and family—and that cuts even deeper.

And I get it. They're the ones who want me to get better the most.

But when I'm told to "exercise more" or "just try this," it feels like they're really saying, "*You're not trying hard enough.*"

You wouldn't tell someone with two broken legs to stand out of their wheelchair and just "try harder."

Trust me—I'm trying. Way more than you realize.

37

I'm not lazy.

Being lazy is choosing to *not* do something.

Me? I'm exhausted, hurting, and walking around with a brain that's basically a clusterf*ck carnival of emotions and dark thoughts I can't shut off.

38

Diet & lifestyle policing.

Yes, I had a piece of cake. No, that doesn't mean I'm not really sick or that I don't care, or that I'm not trying.

It means I'm human. Sometimes I just want to indulge a little without being made to feel guilty about it.

39

"You're too young to be this sick."

Hearing this reinforces the false idea that only the elderly get sick, making it harder for people like me to be taken seriously.

Trust me—I already know I'm too young for this. Saying it back to me only adds to the pain.

40

If you see me dressed nicely and
smiling from ear to ear, it doesn't
erase my illness, and it doesn't make
me a faker or a liar.

I have some good days, some bad
days, and so many in between.

Enjoying myself when I feel good isn't
a crime, and I don't want to be
punished for it with judgment.

HOPE, TREATMENTS & LETDOWNS

41

Just because I'm angry, or bitter, or depressed over my current situation, it doesn't mean I don't constantly hope for a treatment that will make me feel like my old self again.

I do hope.

But I hope cautiously because of how many times I've been let down by the medical system.

42

“Let the doctors figure it out.”

Right. People like me don’t fit into the current medical system. Most doctors don’t understand me or outright don’t believe me.

Do you know how horrible a feeling that is? To be made to feel like it’s *all in my head*?

I *wish* it were all in my head.

43

The hope cycle is like being told every week that you've got great odds of winning the lottery.

At first, you're excited. You believe. You keep hoping.

But after weeks, months—even years—of never winning, you start expecting disappointment every time you buy a damn ticket.

44

Getting a referral to see a new doctor or specialist is a lot like going on a blind date.

You're nervous, hopeful—excited, even. What if this is *the one*?

Spoiler: it's not.

45

You know what's really messed up about chronic illness? I *want* something to be wrong with me.

Sleep apnea? Sure. Some rare disease? Yes, please!

Because a treatable diagnosis means I could go back to being healthy if treatment works. The scariest thing isn't being sick—it's not having any answers, or being told this is my life now and that it's not going to get any better.

46

One of the hardest things about having a chronic illness is when a medical professional makes you feel like you're exaggerating or imagining your symptoms.

When you're told, *That's not normal. You shouldn't be in any pain.* Or, worse, when they prescribe antidepressants or anti-anxiety medication and refer you to a psychologist.

All I want are answers and to feel better—not to be told I'm crazy and that my condition isn't real.

47

When you have a chronic illness, you need to become your own advocate and your own detective, because the medical system isn't designed to help people like me.

Because if you don't fight for yourself, no one else will.

It's honestly exhausting.

48

I've become an expert waiter.

I wait in waiting rooms. I wait for referrals. I wait for test results.

Seriously. If you need any advice on how to wait, just ask.

49

Apparently, stress causes all chronic illnesses. Can you believe that f*cking bull—

Wait, hold on.

I need to manage my stress better so that I can cure myself.

50

On my good days, I actually start to believe that I might be magically cured. That all I needed was proper sleep, or the right vitamin, or the right mindset. And that going forward, I'm going to be *normal* again.

And then the next day comes, and I feel like I'm dying.

Until the cycle starts again.

WAYS TO BE SUPPORTIVE

51

Remember how I said I have to be my own advocate in a medical system that doesn't really get me?

That's why it means so much when a partner or family member comes with me to appointments.

It's not just about another set of ears—it makes me feel less alone, like I actually have backup in the room.

52

Be present without trying to fix me.

I know you want me to be better. To heal. So do I. But sometimes I just need a listening ear. Someone to genuinely care about what I'm going through without asking me if I'd consider trying yoga.

53

Believe me.

That's what I want most of all. To feel heard, believed, and validated.

When you question my pain, it feels like you think I'm lying or exaggerating. And when that doubt comes from someone I love, it cuts the deepest.

54

Help with the little things.

Groceries, tidying, making supper.

On bad days, these tasks can feel like climbing a mountain. When you offer, it tells me you see my struggle and want to lighten my load.

55

Celebrate the good days with me.

They're rare, and they matter. So let's use them to do something fun—something that makes both of us smile.

56

Acknowledge my grief.

Hearing you say, “That must be hard,” really validates what I’m going through. It means you truly see me, and that means more than I can express in words.

57

Please be kind to me on my bad days.

Pain makes me short-tempered sometimes, but your kindness and patience help me feel loved even when I'm at my worst.

58

Don't stop inviting me.

Even if I've declined the last twenty times, it means the world to know you still want me there. When the invitations stop, it feels like you've given up on me—and that hurts more than canceling ever could.

59

Check in without pressure.

Even if I've been quiet for a while, a small message to say you're thinking of me can brighten a very dark day. It reminds me I'm cared for, even in my silence.

60

Please, no guilt.

I already feel awful when I miss celebrations. What helps most is when you say, "It's okay; your health comes first. We'll try again another time."

That kind of understanding means the world to me.

THANK YOU 😊

Thank you so much for taking the time to read this book. I hope these pages gave you a little more understanding of what it's like to have a chronic illness.

It means a lot to me that you took the time to read this, and that you WANT to learn more.

So, thank you <3

www.ingramcontent.com/pod-product-compliance
Lightning Source LLC
Chambersburg PA
CBHW070120030426
42335CB00016B/2213
9781990775659